MILK THISTLE

SILYBUM BENEFITS FOR THE LIVER

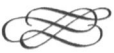

VOYT EDEN

CONTENTS

INTRODUCTION

Milk thistle (Silybummarianum) is a perennial herb with medicinal properties, and the seeds contain silymarin, a group of compounds having antioxidant and anti-inflammatory effects. Milk thistle is usually administered as a home remedy to treat liver problems, with the probability that it will "detoxify" the liver.

Currently, there is inadequate scientific data to ascertain whether or not milk thistle can help the liver. Without the benefit of the doubt, milk thistle doesn't appear to exert a significant effect on liver tissues or liver function.

Milk thistle is also called Saint Mary's thistle, Variegated thistle, and Scotch thistle. In traditional Chinese medicine, milk thistle is called da ji, while the seeds are called shuifeiji.

Health Benefits

Usually, milk thistle is used for liver conditions like hepatitis and cirrhosis. The herb is believed to prevent or treat high cholesterol, diabetes, heartburn or indigestion (dyspepsia), hangover, gallbladder problems, menstrual pain (dysmenorrheal), depression, and even certain types of cancer. Some of these claims have been approved.

Here is what some of the current research says: **Liver Disease**

Some initial studies have suggested that silymarin may improve liver function by keeping toxic substances from binding to liver cells. However, studies on the milk thistle's effectiveness have yielded mixed results in treating liver disorders.

From a comprehensive review of studies in the American Journal of Gastroenterology, milk thistle neither enhances liver function nor lowers the risk of death in people with alcoholic liver disease, hepatitis B, or hepatitis C. Several studies have indicated the benefit of milk thistle for people with mild, subacute (symptom-free) liver disease. An initial study from Finland found that a four-week course of silymarin supplements lowered key liver enzymes in people with a subacute illness, suggesting the liver was functioning normally.

Despite the positive findings, later studies have been unable to replicate the results or demonstrate that the prescription of milk thistle would have the same effects. This book will give you a broad idea about the benefits of milk thistle beyond just the liver.

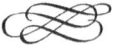

CHAPTER 1

MILK THISTLE

MILK THISTLE IS a natural and safe option for the treatment of many liver-related conditions. Its extract is generally well tolerated, with only rarely-reported, mild side effects, including headaches, stomach upset and nausea.

The herb is used in pregnancy with no toxic effects, however it is advisable to consult your GP before using milk thistle if you are pregnant or nursing. As a general precaution due to its mild oestrogenic effects, people with a history of hormone-related cancers should use milk thistle with caution and under the supervision of a doctor.

The interaction of herbs with some medications should be initially cleared by a medical professional. Consult your

GP to clarify your liver status or health especially if you notice a yellowish color on your skin and eyes, abdominal pain and swelling, itchy skin, coloured urine, chronic fatigue, nausea or vomiting.

HOW TO DETOX WITH MILK THISTLE

THE LIVER HAS regenerative properties in the right environment. Milk thistle shouldn't be seen as general liver treatment; there is enough evidence to support its practical use as a remedy for those who usually over-indulge in fatty foods or alcoholic drinks. Milk thistle helps to detoxify chemicals and toxins that accumulate in the body, accelerates liver-cell regeneration, and improves liver function over time.

It isn't a trend, yet the true extent of its benefits is yet uncovered. The herb is used in several forms; teas, tinctures, capsules or tablets. When buying a milk thistle supplement, look for the Traditional Herbal Registration (THR) logo to ensure that the product is manufactured to a high standard of purity and quality, and has a good concentration of silymarin.

Its long-term use is safe when instructions are followed. However, herbal remedies alone shouldn't be relied on. Milk thistle should be combined with a liver-cleansing diet loaded with garlic, green tea, apples, avocados, olive oil, lemons, and wholegrains for useful results. Also, the intake of fatty, processed and refined foods that place further demands on the liver should be reduced.

In conclusion, drink plenty of water, and avoid excessive toxins from coffee and alcohol. We'd love to hear your experience of using milk thistle for liver detox!

MILK THISTLE AND BREASTFEEDING

MILK THISTLE and breastfeeding have been linked for a very long time. It is a plant of legend called Saint Mary's Thistle and Our Lady's thistle. Historically, it is observed that white veins ran through the leaves of milk thistle when Mary, The Virgin Mother's milk splashed onto the plant. To some, the white veins symbolize breast milk and it is believed to increase breast milk supply when used by a breastfeeding mother.

MILK THISTLE and Breast Milk Supply

BEYOND THE LEGENDS, milk thistle has yielded positive results with breastfeeding mothers in India and Europe for generations. Although no valid scientific proof has beenreported that milk thistle can help a nursing mother make more breast milk, it has been shown to increase milk production in dairy cows. It is believed that the estrogens found in the milk thistle plant could increase breastmilk production as some women have reported thatwhen they take this herb, more breast milk is produced.

How Breastfeeding Women Can Use Milk Thistle to Make More Breast Milk

• MILK THISTLE TEA: tea can be made from the seeds of the milk thistle plant and drank twice to thrice daily. Put a teaspoon of crushed, ground, or chopped milk thistle seeds into 8 ounces (240 ml) of boiling water. Leave to infuse for 10-20 minutes, then enjoy.

• MILK THISTLE SUPPLEMENTS: These come in capsules, soft gels, powder, and a liquid extract which is available online, in health food or vitamin stores. For usage, be sure to buy a herbal supplement from a reputable source and follow all directions for that particular herbal product. You should communicate with your doctor or a lactation consultant for correct information on dosage.

· · ·

• MILK THISTLE AS FOOD: Once the spines are removed, every part of the milk thistle plant is edible. The seeds can be roasted or used for tea; the leaves can be eaten raw or cooked, while the buds can be enjoyed in a similar way to tiny artichokes.

• BREASTFEEDING TEAS AND LACTATION SUPPLEMENTS: Milk thistle is found as a common ingredient in some of the ready-made nursing teas or lactation supplements which are available commercially. It is usually combined with other breastfeeding herbs such as fenugreek, fennel, goat's rue, marshmallow root, and verbena.

HEALTH BENEFITS

• SILYMARIN IS an ingredient found in milk thistle, which helps in repairing the liver cells and rebuild the body.

• MILK THISTLE detoxifies and cleanses the liver.

• IF IT IS TAKEN right after certain types of poisons have been ingested, milk thistle may help prevent liver damage.

. . .

- IT IS beneficial for people with jaundice, cirrhosis or hepatitis since it can reduce the
  swelling of the liver.

- MILK THISTLE MAY HELP LOWER blood sugar levels in people with type 2 diabetes.

- IT IS TAKEN to lower high cholesterol levels.

- IT HAS antioxidant and anticancer properties which help lower the risk of breast, prostate and cervical cancer.

- WHEN CANCER PATIENTS use milk thistle during treatments, the liver and kidneys may be protected from some of the adverse effects of chemotherapy.

WARNINGS AND SIDE Effects

- WHEN PREGNANT OR BREASTFEEDING, always consult your

doctor, a lactation consultant, or a herbal specialist before taking any herbs. Many herbs are similar to medicine and can be harmful if not taken as instructed. There might be interference of herbal benefits when used with other medications.

• BLESSED THISTLE IS AN ENTIRELY different plant and should not be confused with milk thistle.

• THERE ARE reports of rare allergic reactions to milk thistle. If you are allergic to ragweed, daisies, marigolds, or chrysan-themums, do not use milk thistle. It belongs to the same plant family.

• MILK THISTLE IS GENERALLY a safe herb whose most common side effects are considered mild and stomach related. When taken excessively, it leads to loose bowel movements, stomach upset, nausea, and vomiting.

• AMONG THE USES of milk thistle are liver cleansing and body detoxification. During the cleansing process, toxins are released from the internal system into the bloodstream for removal. When these toxins are present in the blood, they can enter the breast milk and be transferred to the baby. If toxins from heavy smoking, alcohol, or the use of drugs are stored in your liver, beware of milk thistle while you're breastfeeding.

• BEWARE OF MILK thistle while using seizure medication Dilantin (phenytoin).

• MILK THISTLE interference with birth control pills can make them less effective. Also, problems can arise if you're taking antipsychotic or antianxiety drugs,
    certain cancer medications, or blood thinners. Inform your doctor about any medication, before the use of milk thistle.

OTHER WAYS TO Increase Your Supply

MILK THISTLE, as well as other breastfeeding herbs, tends to help some women increase low milk supply. Nevertheless, this treatment does not work for everyone. Other actions you can take to stimulate your body and help improve your breast milk supply include breastfeeding more often, breastfeeding for a more extended period at each feeding, and using a breast pump after or between breast-feedings.

WHEN TO SEEK Help

IF YOU HAVE a low breast milk supply, and the natural and herbal treatments don't help, it's time to seek help. Consult your doctor or a lactation consultant. The faster the problem is detected, the quicker the issue can be fixed and you can get back to breastfeeding successfully.

THE CONNECTION between Milk Thistle and Liver Care

OVER THE YEARS, you've probably come across articles that talks about the importance of the liver to the body. The liver is no doubt a vital organ of the body which has different functions such as detoxification, protein synthesis and the production of biochemical aids which help digestion. To survive you need the liver. It's a well-known fact that a human can only survive 24 hours without a proper and functioning liver. Liver diseases can be defined as infections that affect the liver. Examples of these diseases include cancer, hepatitis, glycogen storage disease type II, etc. These diseases are quite harmful and have highly damaging capacities.

Liver infection also has external signs such as excessive sweating, coated tongue, skin rashes, bad breath, itchy skin and eyes, offensive body odor, blemishes on the skin, acne, dark circles under the eyes, brownish spots and flushed facial appearance or excessive facial blood vessels.

Other symptoms include easy bleeding, pale stools, bone loss, dark urine, itching, small, enlarged spleen, spider-like blood vessels visible in the skin, pain from the biliary tract or pancreas and an enlarged gallbladder. These might sound orlook scary but don't worry:. ccience and Mother Nature have provided solutions to these ailments. A few years ago people were not aware of the natural potential and effectiveness of the herb called Milk Thistle for liver care. This is a plant that has a branched and crumpled stem with milky white veins. These veins produce a white-colour fluid, which is the main reason it is named that way.

THERE ARE few natural remedial herbs which are used for treatment of the liver. These are Oregon grape root, milk thistle, licorice root, dandelion root, astragalus, yellow dock, chicory root, golden seal, licorice and turmeric. However, milk thistle and liver care are the perfect match. Milk Thistle and liver care have long formed a great partnership.

Silymarin forms a significant ingredient in these plants

which serves as an anti-oxidant and helps the liver to fight germs, viruses or bacteria in the human body. It also helps in protecting the liver against harmful toxins released by external agents. It also protects the liver against poisons.

MILK THISTLE and liver care is an important topic in the medical research field. One great method of keeping your liver healthy is referred to as 'liver flushing'. This can always be used an hour before meals or drugs. Have a cup of lemon juice or grapefruit mix with two cloves, fresh pressed garlic and a tablespoon of olive oil. This will help flush out the toxins from your body hence keep your liver happy and healthy!

CHAPTER 2

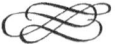

$\mathcal{S}$ UPPLEMENTING WITH MILK THISTLE

THERE ARE many ways in which milk thistle can be incorpo-
rated into your daily diet. Milk thistle seeds and leaves can
be ingested either in pill, powder, tincture, extract, or tea
form.

As a body detoxification process, the recommended daily
intake of milk thistle extract is 450-600 milligrams, sepa-
rated into two or three doses, taken for several months. This
is not the daily required quantity for everyone but can act as
a natural liver "detox." For continuous use and general liver
support, use 150 milligrams daily.

A high-quality product between 150 to 250 milligrams of
milk thistle extract per capsule is recommended, so the

quantity consumed can be adjusted depending on your requirements. You should also look for standardized products that contain at least 80% silymarin. Silymarin is a phytonutrient present in milk thistle, which makes it one of the best nutrients to support liver health and daily

detoxification. Your liver works hard to ensure the smooth running of metabolic processes and free the body from harmful toxins. Today, it's easy for this vital organ to become overwhelmed and choked. Find time to give it a little extra support with milk thistle.

GENERAL LIVER DETOXIFICATION

WITHOUT A DOUBT, milk thistle is a potent liver cleanser that helps to remove toxins from the body. It repairs damaged liver cells by bringing them back to a functional and healthy state. Milk thistle can naturally reverse the damaging effects of many harmful—yet familiar— substances, like alcohol, sugar, pesticides in the food supply, heavy metals in the water supply, and pollution in the air. Liver damage caused by acetaminophen, as well as chemotherapy, radiation, and some poisonous mushrooms can also be reduced.

The health of the body's blood is much dependent on liver health, which is another reason to realise the importance of optimal liver function. As a blood purifier, the liver actively cleans the blood around-the-clock to support every system in our bodies. By helping in liver detoxification, milk thistle naturally helps in this essential blood purification process.

Finally, milk thistle has been proven to restore and maintain glutathione levels in the liver. Glutathione is the body's most powerful endogenous antioxidant and plays a myriad of essential roles in health, including supporting regular detoxification.

HOW LONG BEFORE MILK THISTLE WORKS FOR SKIN

YOU MIGHT THINK that silymarin is a quick cure, use it once, and the body is all better. However that is not necessarily the case.

If you are fighting off a viral infection, a common cold or a flu bug, silymarin provides immune system support and could speed up your recovery. Cold symptoms can last for up to three weeks, but most people can fight off the bug in 7-10 days, without help.

Chronic viral infections, such as hepatitis C, are conditions for which silymarin is often recommended. Prescription drugs are mostly ineffective against viruses. So, alternative solutions are necessary. Alternative practitioners might recommend the dietary supplement for inflammatory conditions, such as arthritis or an inflamed bowel, but there are more effective natural anti-inflammatories. Mainstream practitioners typically stick with the anti-inflammatory drugs, because of their proven effectiveness.

The biggest problem with anti-inflammatory drugs and other prescription medications is that they are hard on the liver. Most over-the-counter and prescription pain relievers now carry warnings about the possibility of liver damage, with prolonged use.

Silymarin is known to support liver health and function. It is now recommended to help protect the liver from toxic drugs. But how long does it take for milk thistle to work to protect or heal the liver?

In one studyworkers exposed to toluene and other toxic substances were given a concentrated silymarin extract for four weeks. There was a significant improvement in liver function tests after that trial period. The researchers recommended that the workers kept taking the supplement, for as long as they continued to be exposed to the toxin.

Because of the benefits to the liver, silymarin is sometimes recommended as a hangover remedy. It's also an ingredient in some energy drinks on the market. How long does it take for milk thistle to begin to relieve a hangover?

There's not much scientific information to support the use of the botanical for that purpose. Whether or not it will improve a person's energy levels remains to be seen. The effect is likely to vary from one person to the next.

Other factors that can affect the length of time before milk thistle works include a person's overall health and nutritional intake. A person that eats well and gets good nutritional support from dietary supplements should see results quickly. It might take a little longer for someone who is in poor health, eats terrible food or is poorly nourished.

The speed of recovery will also depend on the quality of the supplement being taken. If it is a concentrated extract, it will work faster than ground seeds. The silymarin concentration should be listed on the label of ingredients.

To have the healthiest liver, it is important to avoid things that are toxic to it. Avoiding foods containing chemical additives and skincare products containing synthetic ingredients will help.

So really, how long does it take for milk thistle to work to improve the skin's appearance? Although the anti-inflammatory activity is beneficial for many skin conditions, you need to use good skin care products, too, if you want to see results.

How to Cure Erectile Dysfunction at Home

ERECTILE DYSFUNCTION (IMPOTENCE) can be quite embarrassingbut curable. Many medicinal and natural remedies are available to get you back to form in no time. Here are some home remedies that can assist you to cure erectile dysfunction. Some of these ideas are yet to be evaluated by the Food and Drug Administration; therefore, it is advisable to see a doctor regarding any dietary changes.

• USE OF ALLIUM sativum or garlic as a potent remedy for treating erectile dysfunction. Chinese and Indian physicians have used it as an aphrodisiac for many years. Combine one tablespoonful of garlic with one tablespoonful of honey three times daily. Carrots are believed to combat impotence, especially when combined with warm milk. This can lead to an improvement in your dysfunction.

• TAKE A CUP OF SEASONED RAISINS, a cup of prunes, a cup of walnuts, a cup of dried apricots and two full lemons and blend them all at once with a few tablespoons of honey. This is known to be an old-wives'-tale type mixture that may help if a teaspoonful is taken three times per day, at least thirty minutes before mealtimes. Onion has been touted as second only to garlic for enhancing sexual health. Try to make one hundred milliliters of the extract three times a day.

It is apparent that smokers are liable to die young, so quit smoking. Make an honest assessment of the choices that affect your health and wellness. For instance, smoking can also inhibit a man's ability to achieve and maintain an erection in addition to causing a myriad of health issues, according to the Centers for Disease Control. If you smoke, quitting should be your first and most important step toward a natural erectile dysfunction cure. Life is often determined by the decisions we make and the priorities we set. Be honest with yourself about what is more important to you, and the truth shall set you free.

You can also use remedies involving Indian herbs to cure erectile dysfunction. Herbs that can only be found in specialty stores are often mentioned by the Indian Ayurvedic treatment of conditions. Here are some Ayurvedic treatments to cure impotence. In the morning try to take an equal portion of powdered acacia seedless pods and unrefined sugar and take six grams with a glass of milk. Honey, milk and an infusion of jambul fruit may help you to get rid of erectile dysfunction. Finally, fifty grams of dried Indian gooseberry with fifty grams of mango ginger and one hundred grams of unrefined sugar should be mixed with milk as an early morning libido enhancer.

Many things lead to erectile dysfunction, many of which may be influenced by herbal remedies. Poor circulation may contribute to impotence problems, in which case Ginkgo biloba is a well-known cure. Yohimbe, an African herb, can aid your staying power and ginseng is believed to enhance testosterone levels. Milk thistle and schizandra can help to rebuild your damaged internal organ if alcoholic beverages have limited your sexual capacity. Stress can also lead to impotence. Kava and valerian are two herbs that you can use to get rid of the problem. It is essential to watch prescription drugs that may be leading to your condition. Try to change or replace the drugs with more natural treatments that may not have the same sexual side effects.

THE NATURAL WAY To Beat Psoriasis

A SIGNIFICANT CONCERN for all individuals are skin problems, since they can look ugly. . Psoriasis is a skin condition that needs cautious observation. If you are affected with psoriasis, your skin breaks out with itchy rashes, white flakes, and unwanted blemishes.

HOW DOES PSORIASIS DEVELOP?

IF YOU HAVE PSORIASIS, your skin cells automatically multiply at such a quick pace, that the rashes develop at once. Healthy skin will renew itself over a period of 30 days. However, the infected cells in psoriasis-affected skin move from the inner-most part of the skin layer to the top surface in about three days. The result is an itchy and reddish rash on the skin. More so, as the cells accumulate on tthe topmost layer of the skin, they eventually die and dry off, then becoming flaky and whitish.

How can psoriasis be cured?

SADLY, psoriasis has a natural remedy but it appears to be presently incurable. Most doctors and dermatologists are yet to uncover the causative agent. You can try these natural psoriasis treatments below at anytime.

Once in a while, expose your skin to the sun's heat. The early morning sun's temperature assists the body in the development of vitamin D which fights off psoriasis in you. The UVB rays provide better skin treatment but may cause sunburn. In this case, it is best to apply some sunscreen protection to the skin parts not affected by psoriasis.

Drink teas. Take in sarsaparilla capsules, nettle leaves, or milk thistle. Take in flaxseed or fish oil regularly. You can begin taking in a dose of 1500 mg of fish oil a day.

Use some granular lecithin placed on a tablespoon. You may incorporate them with the cereal you eat in the morning, with your salad or soup, or in smoothies. It is not recommended to add the granular lecithin to boiling water or for it to be used as cooking oil.

Take in large quantities of vitamin B in the form of inositol. To lessen the itchy sensation, apply diluted apple cider vinegar on the affected area.

Many people in the world have Psoriasis. Psoriasis is a complicated disease that attacks a small part of the population, there are many different medicines and treatments for the disease, but many keep looking for a 'natural' Psoriasis treatment.

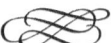

CHAPTER 3

*H*ERBAL REMEDIES FOR LIVER HEALTH

Chronic Hepatitis C

MILK THISTLE IS SELDOM USED by people with chronic hepatitis C (a viral infection characterized by the progressive scarring of the liver). As reported by a survey conducted by the National Institutes of Health, 23% of 1,145 hepatitis C patients used herbal supplements with milk thistle being the commonest.

The survey reported that when taking milk thistle, people with hepatitis C had fewer symptoms and a "somewhat better quality of life" despite having no measurable change in viral activity or liver inflammation.

A Journal of the American Medical Association (JAMA) published in 2012 confirmed this. Silymarin, despite being well-tolerated in the study (prescribed three times daily in 420 or 700-milligram doses) had no real effect on liver enzymes.

DESPITE THESE CONTRADICTIONS, many scientists believe that milk thistle delivers something of a placebo effect in which a person feels there is an improvement in symptoms despite having no change in their clinical condition.

Type 2 Diabetes

SEVERAL STUDIES HAVE SUGGESTED the benefits of milk thistle for people with diabetes especially type 2 diabetes.

According to research published in Phytomedicine in 2015, silymarin used in a 45-day plan increased antioxidant capacity and generally reduced inflammation in adults with type 2 diabetes better than a placebo.

According to the author's study, findings suggested that silymarin may reduce the oxidative stress commonly associated with diabetes complications.

. . .

In 2016, a consistent review further concluded that the daily use of silymarin appears to reduce high blood glucose and HbA1C levels, although the authors warned that the quality of the reviewed studies was poor.

Possible Side Effects

Some side effects triggered by milk thistle include headache, nausea, diarrhea, abdominal bloating, and gas. Less severely, muscle aches, joint pain, and sexual dysfunction.

Allergic reactions are also possible. People allergic to ragweed, daisies, artichokes, kiwi, or plants in the aster family may also be allergic to milk thistle. Seldomly, milk thistle can cause a potentially life-threatening, all-body allergy known as anaphylaxis and if not treated, can cause shock, coma, cardiac or respiratory failure, or death.

Drug Interaction

Milk thistle needs to be used with caution as it may trigger hypoglycemia (low blood sugar) in people on diabetes medications.

Milk thistle and the supplement should be avoided by people in hormone-sensitive states like endometriosis, uterine fibroids, breast, uterus and ovary-cancer sufferers, because it exerts a mild estrogen-like effect. It may also reduce the effectiveness of estrogen-based contraceptives.

Milk thistle can alter the way that your body metabolizes certain drugs in the liver, triggering interactions with:

• ANTIBIOTICS LIKE BIAXIN (clarithromycin)

• ANTICOAGULANTS LIKE COUMADIN (warfarin)

• NON-STEROIDAL ANTI-INFLAMMATORY DRUGS (NSAIDs) like Advil (ibuprofen), Celebrex (celecoxib), and Voltaren (diclofenac)

• STATIN DRUGS like Mevacor (lovastatin) and Lescol (fluvastatin), etc.

To avoid complications, seek your doctor's advice on any supplements or herbal remedies you are taking.

. . .

Dosage and Preparation

NO GUIDELINES EXIST DIRECTING the appropriate use of milk thistle. Milk thistle supplements are commonly sold in capsule form but are also available as tablets, tea bags, and oral tinctures. Doses vary from 175 milligrams to 1,000 milligrams and the higher the dose, the greater the risk of side effects.

Combined remedies like Iberogast drops (used to treat dyspepsia) and Barberol tablets (formulated for diabetics) are considered potent with milk thistle in doses of 10 pg. 35 milligrams and 210 milligrams, respectively. Higher dosage does not equate to better results.

Dietary supplements of milk thistle are sold in natural foods stores, pharmacies, stores that specialize in herbal products and online stores.

What to Look For

NO RIGOROUS TESTING and research is needed for dietary supplements in the United States compared to pharmaceutical drugs. This has led to variations in the quality of the supplement.

Select products that have undergone testing and certification by an independent certifying body like the U.S. Pharmacopeia (USP), ConsumerLab, and NSF International for safety and quality. Besides, opt for brands that have been organically certified under the regulations of the U.S. Department of Agriculture (USDA).

Two-Phase Process of Milk Thistle That Suppresses Cellular Inflammation

MILK THISTLE'S anti-inflammatory effect is one of the best, and research also suggests that there can be a two-phase process that is similar to other beneficial natural compounds such as curcumin which can be found in turmeric and EGCG commonly known as Epigallocatechin gallate a component of green tea. According to research the first-phase cellular response to silymarin in cells is a rapid increase in the expression of genes that are associated with cellular stress, and to be specific endoplasmic reticulum (ER). In some certain cases, such stress may lead to death.

The second phase includes a much longer suppression of gene expression which is associated with inflammation and also inhibiting inflammation, as well as:

. . .

• ACTIVATING AMP-ACTIVATED PROTEIN KINASE (AMPK) — AMPK is an enzyme that can be found in your body's cells. It can sometimes be called the "metabolic master switch" because it plays a vital role in regulating metabolism. "AMPK helps in the induction of events within cells involved in maintaining energy homeostasis. "AMPK helps in the regulation of various biological activities that balance the glucose, lipid and energy imbalances. Metabolic syndrome (Mets) becomes effective when the AMPK- regulated pathways are turned off which triggers a syndrome such as energy imbalances, hyperglycemia, and lipid abnormalities.

AMPK ALSO CONTROLS the response to these stressors, shifts energy toward cellular repair, maintains or helps in returning to homeostasis and increases the likelihood of survival. Adiponectin and hormones leptin aids AMPK. To summarise this, Activating AMPK also produces the same benefits as dieting, weight loss, and exercise. This can be considered beneficial for maladies."

• INHIBITING mammalian target of rapamycin (mTOR) is beneficial when the mTOR pathway is activated which may increase the risk of cancer. There is a high possibility that most doctors are not taught this in the medical school and the majority of ~~hmm~~ them are not aware of it. There are several doctors that have been targeted to utilize this pathway. These same pathways drugs have also been tested on animals towards extending their lifespan.

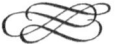

CHAPTER 4

ILK THISTLE BEYOND YOUR LIVER

MILK THISTLE no doubt contains silymarin and silybin antioxidants which are commonly known to protect the liver from toxins and the effect of alcohol. Silymarin has been found to increase glutathione which is a powerful antioxidant that is vital for liver detoxification and it also regenerates liver cells. , However, it would be unfair to see milk thistle only as an a herb for liver health. Milk Thistle has numerous benefits. Among these benefits are its anti-cancerous effects, which have been recommended by the American Botanical Council

Several studies, both in vitro and in vivo, suggest that milk thistle can be used to treat or prevent different cancers;

increasing apoptosis and inhibiting prostate cancer, inhibiting and stimulating the regression of skin tumors with topical applications, inhibiting the induction of tongue squamous-cell cancer; inhibiting growth and DNA synthesis in breast and cervical cancer cells, decreasing incidences of bladder neoplasms, inhibiting proliferation in leukemia cells and reducing the frequency of drug-induced colon adenocarcinomas.

Silybin is effective and useful against hormone-refractory prostate cancer and also aids the efficacy of tumor necrosis factor TNF-alpha-based chemotherapy. It's a well-known fact that its liver-protectant effects in chemo and radiation therapies will offer more value to cancer patients as milk thistle's antineoplastic effects work well especially for drug-resistant cancers. Milk thistle and omega-3 fatty acids used before radiation enhance the survival times and deliver fewer side effects in patients with metastasizing brain tumors. According to some pharmacological studies, topic silymarin is as beneficial as sunscreens in protecting against ultraviolet-B-induced skin cancers.

4 MORE POTENTIAL HEALTH BENEFITS OF MILK THISTLE

MILK THISTLE PROVIDES other benefits as well, such as:

. . .

• KIDNEY HEALTH —Milk thistle has relatively similar effects on the kidneys as on the liver. It aids in stimulating cell
pg. 41
regeneration in the kidneys and can be useful in the patient's dialysis.

• HEART HEALTH — Milk thistle raises the levels and the benefit of HDL cholesterol and reduces the risk of atherosclerosis.

• DIABETES — Silymarin improves glycemia and also decreases glycosylated hemoglobin, total cholesterol, fasting blood glucose, triglycerides, and LDL cholesterol. Milk thistle helps in the improvement of blood sugar control in people living with diabetes.

• BRAIN HEALTH — It said that milk thistle has neuroprotective properties which might be beneficial for several sclerosis and Parkinson's disease. According to animal studies it has been stated that silymarin suppresses the formation of amyloid beta protein: a toxic protein that is linked to Alzheimer's, helping reduce Alzheimer's disease.

VOYT EDEN

To add to these features, milk thistle is safer and can be used by many people with little or no side effects.

Generally, milk thistle has been identified as one of the safest and best-tolerated herbs with limited side effects. However, no short-term trials of high silymarin intake have been carried out in a healthy population. Milk thistle is safe and has an oral standard that contains 70 or 80 percent silymarin at a dosage of 420mg.

If you have any challenges or you have any strange feelings regarding your kidneys or liver, or you're interested in any of the potential antidiabetic, anticancer and heart-boosting properties of silymarin, the best thing for you would be a milk thistle supplement. If you're dieting, you can as well find silymarin in turmeric, artichokes, and coriander (cilantro), however, milk thistle has been proven to be the richest known source.

CONSIDERATIONS BEFORE GROWING MILK THISTLE AT HOME

YOU NEED to be careful before planting milk thistle in your garden. It's a highly invasive weed that spreads and could well spread across the lawn and the neighborhood. Milk thistle can be toxic to livestock and animals roaming your yard, and you should endeavor not to plant it outdoors. Milk thistle has the potential to grow in any soil, even poor-quality soil. If you're considering growing milk thistle, you need to plant the seeds at least a quarter-inch deep after the last frost. It is best to place them where they can be fully exposed to the sun. Once ythe flowers have started to dry and a white pappus tuff begins to form, they are ready for harvest.

How to Store **Milk Thistle**

STORING milk thistle isn't that complex; all you need to do is to place the flower heads in a paper bag and keep it in a dry and cool place. This will enable the drying process to continue and once you're sure they are well dried, give the bag a few whacks as this will enable you to separate the seeds from the flowers heads, "Milk thistle is best when it is placed in a dry and airtight container. Take it out only when you're about to use it.

CAN YOU GROW MILK THISTLE?

MILK THISTLE IS a vigorous plant that grows well in diverse environments, preferably high temperatures, dry conditions, and well-drained soil. To plant milk thistle, scatter the seeds over the loose soil in the spring or fall as it takes around two weeks to germinate. Space each seed cluster about 12 inches apart because it grows in clumps. Milk thistle is drought-resistant and needs minimal watering.

Once the flowers have completed blooming, seed clusters will be left behind which can be harvested and the seed extracted by removing the fluffy fibers surrounding it. The seeds can be air-dried or you can use a home dehydrator (which lowers the risk of fungal contamination).

The seeds can be ground into powder using mortar and pestle, once dried. Milk thistle tonic is usually made by infusing a tablespoon of ground seed in three cups of hot water for 20 minutes

Never harvest milk thistle plants exposed to pesticides or found along roadways or industrial sites.

How Strong Is the Evidence?

MILK THISTLE HAS BEEN WELL STUDIED and analyzed, with over

200 clinical studies conducted over the last 30 years. However, some of these studies are poorly designed, and liver regeneration is a slow process, making it difficult to test. The confirmation for alcoholic and non-alcoholic liver

disease is relatively stable, while it is mixed for other conditions:

• ALCOHOLIC RELATED LIVER DISEASE (ARLD): Excessive alcohol consumption is the main cause of liver damage and disease, especially alcoholic fatty liver disease, alcoholic hepatitis, and cirrhosis. There is much evidence showing that milk thistle improves liver function and may increase survival in some patients. The herb's anti-fibrotic properties help to prevent liver tissue scarring and counter the negative effects of alcohol consumption. In some European countries, including Germany, milk thistle is now recommended by doctors to treat alcoholic- related liver disease.

• NON-ALCOHOLIC LIVER DISEASE (NAFLD): Accumulation of fat is primarily due to a

combination of high-fat, high-carbohydrate diets and sedentary lifestyles are the primary cause of liver damage. Non-alcoholic liver disease is now estimated to affect 25%-30% of the adult UK population. If detected early, a build-up of fat within liver cells can be reversed, but if left untreated, inflammation, fibrosis, hepatitis, and cirrhosis can be triggered. A study compared the effectiveness of silymarin (140mg) against the widely-used liver medications metformin and pioglitazone. Findings revealed that participants in the silymarin group had the most significant blood levels of liver enzymes reduced, suggesting that it offered greater protection against liver damage.

• LIVER CANCER: Mixed findings observed that milk thistle potentially has some anti-cancerous effects. Several large-scale studies found that milk thistle can improve liver function and reduce the risk of mortality in patients with liver cancer. However, milk thistle has not yet been proven effective as an anti-cancer therapy in humans. Researchers are 'optimistically cautious' about its potential as studies have seen little to no benefits.

• CHEMOTHERAPY AND MEDICATION PRESCRIPTION: Initial evidence suggests that milk thistle may improve the effectiveness of certain chemotherapy drugs targeted at ovarian and breast cancer, including cisplatin and doxorubicin. Chemotherapy and medication prescriptions contain toxins that are broken down in the liver, where they often activate inflammation. Milk thistle may help to regenerate liver cells damaged by these substances and lower the adverse results of chemotherapy on the liver without reducing its effectiveness. However, the evidence is hindered by poor study methods. Therefore, reliable clinical trials are required

• • •

- HANGOVERS: Milk thistle is known to aid liver recovery from alcohol, many people consume milk thistle before and after drinking to lessen the severity of the subsequent hangover. The herb remains the go-to hangover elimination technique despite little clinical evidence to back it up.

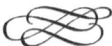

CHAPTER 5

*B*ENEFITS AND MILK THISTLE SEED SMOOTHIE RECIPE

IF YOU LOVE EXPLORING new superfoods, you will love this recipe. Milk Thistle is often recommended to help with liver and gallbladder disorders.

MILK THISTLE SEED History

THE PRICKLY MILK thistle has been in existence and used for over 2,000years as a herbal remedy. A native plant of the Mediterranean region it is often used in both food and medicine. However, we can now find this same plant across the globe being grown in dry, sunny areas.

What is Milk Thistle Seed?

Milk thistle contains the antioxidant silymarin, which helps to support liver health and hormonal balance.

Our liver filters out the toxins our body absorbs, and this includes excess hormones. Milk thistle seed helps in stimulating the liver to cleanse itself, as well as stimulating the renewal of liver cells and stimulating the liver and gallbladder to secrete bile which helps in digestion.

Add milk thistle seed to your smoothie, the combination is superb, as it is effective yet with a mild flavor. One good thing about this is that you have a tasty smoothie and at the same time protect your liver.

MILK THISTLE SEED BLUEBERRY SMOOTHIE RECIPE

• 1/2 cup frozen blueberries

• 1 large frozen banana

. . .

- 1 TSP MACA POWDER

- 1 TSP MILK Thistle Seed Powder

- 1 TSP CHIA Seeds

- 1/2 WATER or nut milk

- A HANDFUL of fresh mint leaves

ADD and mix everything in your blender. If preferred you can also add blueberries. Freeze the blueberries and banana to give the smoothie a creamy chilled texture. This is perfect for your breakfast

As said earlier Milk Thistle Seed powder has a mild taste, and so it's quite easy to add it to soups and smoothies as a thickener.

YOU CAN ALSO USE maca powder because it helps to balance

your hormones, so it is perfect for those that have hormonal issues.

USE IT FOR DETOXING!

MILK THISTLE also helps in parasite cleansing. This is so effective because, silymarin is the primary component in Milk thistle which helps in the removal of liver toxins.

Toxins are powerful and accumulate in the liver for most people who drink alcohol, who are stressed or hardly ever eat good food. Milk Thistle helps in cleansing the toxins which are given off by parasites. It also aids liver-cell regeneration, and its antioxidant action helps in protecting against cell damage from toxins.

Other interesting Milk Thistle Facts

1. Traditionally Milk Thistle has contributed to an increase in breastmilk production

2. It helps to save or prevent people from Death Cap mushroom poisoning

3. It is used to protect and heal the livers of people who have undergone chemotherapy

. . .

PRECAUTIONS: You need to consult your doctors if you're on any medications or taking some forms of oral contraceptives.

9 AMAZING HEALTH FACT MILK THISTLE FOR SKIN, HAIR, HEALTH.

- PREVENTS ACNE, Eczema
  - purifies
  - prevents skin cancer and photo-aging
  - protects hair follicles
  - prevents hair loss:
  treats liver problems

8 BENEFITS of Milk Thistle Tea

THE MOST SIGNIFICANT health benefits of milk thistle tea include healing the liver, lowering cholesterol levels, soothing inflammation, improving digestion, and detoxifying the body. It also helps in regulating blood-sugar levels and prevents chronic disease.

Milk Thistle tea is made with powdered seeds, crushed from the milk thistle plant and its scientific name is Silybum marianum. The name 'milk thistle' was coined from the milky discharge that comes out after crushing the flowers of the plant.

Milk Thistle has been used for traditional medicines for

THOUSANDS OF YEARS because of the powerful active ingredients in the flower and seeds and it's one of the most common choices for natural health practitioners.

HEALTH BENEFITS of Milk Thistle Tea

MILK THISTLE tea is specifically effective for people suffering from diabetes, arthritis, indigestion, anxiety or obesity. This is quite powerful because of its active ingredient silymarin, and also antioxidants, vitamins, and minerals.

TREATS LIVER Cirrhosis

THE LIVER IS one of the most complex organs to heal or repair; this is why liver cirrhosis and other conditions affecting the liver can be very critical to health. Silymarin is the active ingredient in milk thistle tea, it is composed of three different flavonoids and is directly linked to repairing liver cells and helps the recovery process of liver disease patients.

Reduces Inflammation

MILK THISTLE tea has some anti-inflammatory properties that help ease the pain of arthritis, headaches, gout, migraines, joint disorders, aches and stomach upset etc.

PROTECTS HEART HEALTH

MILK THISTLE tea is commonly known to reduce blood pressure and cholesterol, which relieves stress on the cardiovascular system. This can lower your risk of heart attacks, atherosclerosis, and strokes and also coronary heart diseases.

WEIGHT LOSS

SOME WEIGHT LOSS specialists recommend milk thistle tea for people trying to lose weight. It stimulates the metabolism and suppresses the appetite, which increases passive fat-burning and helps people resist snacking in between meals.

Reduces Digestive Issues

People who suffer from cramping, constipation, excess flatulence or bloating can use milk thistle to optimize their digestive system, ensure proper nutrient uptake and relieve inflammation on the gut tissues.

How to make Milk Thistle Tea?

Preparing milk thistle is very simple and can be done in various ways, either as a pure tea, or combining with ingredients or other herbal teas. Some people feel milk thistle has an unpleasant taste, so many prefer sweeteners or herbal combinations.

Milk Thistle Tea

Firstly, you need to decide if you want to use of milk thistle seeds or milk thistle extract. If you're using extract, all you need to do is add 20 drops to a cup of hot water. It is best to drink this tea before meals to aid digestion.

Ingredients

1 TABLESPOON of milk thistle seeds 2 cups of filtered water 1 teaspoon of organic honey, if desired Recipe

• STEP 1: Fill a tea bag with the powdered milk thistle seeds.

• STEP 2: Allow the water to boil and then reduce heat to a simmer.

• STEP 3: Pour the hot water onto the tea bag in a cup and allow it to infuse for 3-5 minutes.

• STEP 4: Add the honey or flavor after removing the tea bag and enjoy!

MILK THISTLE COFFEE

. . .

IF YOU'RE CONSIDERING a different beverage, milk thistle coffee is also a great option.

INGREDIENTS

1 TABLESPOON of powdered milk thistle powdered seeds

1 TABLESPOON of roasted powdered chicory root

1 TABLESPOON of roasted powdered dandelion root 2 cups of filtered water

1 TEASPOON OF SUGAR, if desired Recipe

• STEP 1: Add the milk thistle, chicory root anddandelion root to a French press

• STEP 2: boil water and then add to the French press.

· · ·

- STEP 3: Stir and allow the mixture to steep for 10-15 minutes.

- STEP 4: Depress the French press and pour out the coffee.

- STEP 5: Add sweetener, if you desire. Enjoy!

SIDE EFFECTS of Milk Thistle Tea

MILK THISTLE tea can have a number of side effects, such as:

- BLOATING

- HEARTBURN

- SKIN RASHES

- SWEATING

. . .

- IRRITABILITY

- Insomnia

- Gastrointestinal distress

- VOMITING AND OVERALL WEAKNESS.

- Constipation

Risks

THESE CAN BE EXPERIENCED by people who are allergic to milk thistle, and this can be quite severe. The common side effects are stomach upset and inflammation of the gut.

- Pregnant women: some have argued that drinking milk tea during pregnancy and breastfeeding does not have any side effects. However, you need to be careful what you consume during pregnancy.

- People with diabetes: Because of the sugar-lowering properties of this tea, it can be quite critical for people with diabetes who are already on medication to lower their blood sugar. Using this treatment simultaneously can cause blood-sugar to fall dangerous levels.

• DRUG INTERACTIONS: Milk thistle tea has various active ingredients that interact with drugs and sleep aids, disorders such as diabetes and hypertension and liver disease.

MILK THISTLE OIL

MILK THISTLE IS SOMETIMES ADDED to cosmeticsTo use milk thistle oil for hair, m add one drop of milk thistle oil to 10 drops of your carrier oil and massage it onto your scalp and leave it for 10 minutes before bath time and then rinse and style.

CONCLUSION

IT IS evident from the results that the milk thistle (Silybummarianum) plant has powerful potential to control chemically induced diabetes mellitus in animals and reverse diabetes in animals to a normal condition. Therefore, further studies are required to ascertain and establish a similar effect on other animals. Pharmacological research is necessary to learn the pharmaco-kinetics & dynamics of the drug, which would help the research community in better understanding the impact of the drug so that such an effective drug could be used to treat diabetes on Human subjects as well.

There have been few human studies of milk thistle on liver disease. Promising data has been reported, but some study results are at this time mixed.

Nonetheless studies conducted outside the United States support claims of oral milk thistle improving liver function, despite the flaws in study design and reporting. Presently, no absolute proof regarding its claimed uses is

AVAILABLE. NCCAM wants to better understand the purpose of milk thistle for chronic hepatitis C by supporting phase II research. With the National Institute of Diabetes, Digestive and Kidney Diseases, NCCAM plans further studies of milk thistle for chronic hepatitis C and non-alcoholic steatohepatitis (liver disease that occurs in people who drink little or no alcohol).

Milk thistle is being studied by the National Cancer Institute and the National Institute of Nursing Research, for cancer prevention and to treat complications in HIV patients.

.   .   .

DISCLAIMER

THIS DOCUMENT IS GEARED towards providing exact and reliable information with regards to the topic and issue covered. The publication is sold on the idea that the publisher is not required to hold himself accountable, , officially permitted, or provider of qualified services. If advice is necessary, be it legal or professional, a practiced individual in the profession should be consulted.

- From a Declaration of Principles which was accepted and approved equally by a Committee of the American Bar Association and a Committee of Publishers and Associations.

In no way is it legal to reproduce, duplicate, or transmit any part of this document by either electronic means or in printed format. Recording of this publication is strictly prohibited, and any storage of this document is not allowed unless with written permission from the publisher. All rights reserved.

The information provided herein is stated to be truthful and consistent, in that any liability, regarding inattention or otherwise, by any usage or abuse of any policies, processes, or directions contained within is the solitary and utter responsibility of the recipient reader. Under no circumstances will any legal responsibility or blame be held against the publisher for any reparation, damages, or monetary loss due to the information herein, either directly or indirectly.

Respective authors own all copyrights not held by the publisher.

The information herein is offered for informational purposes solely and is universal as so.

The presentation of the information is without a contract or any guarantee assurance.

The trademarks that are used are without any consent, and the publication of the trademark is without permission or backing by the trademark owner. All trademarks and brands within this book are for clarifying purposes only and are owned by the owners themselves, not affiliated with this document.

www.ingramcontent.com/pod-product-compliance
Lightning Source LLC
Chambersburg PA
CBHW020329290526
45785CB00007B/2982